Epigenetics. The DNA of the Pregnant Mother

ה"ב

EPIGENETICS. THE DNA OF THE PREGNANT MOTHER

HOW TO STRENGHT YOUR GENES AND CREATE SUPER BABIES CONCEIVED NATURALLY OR BY EGG DONATION

"Every great journey begins with a first step".Lao Tse

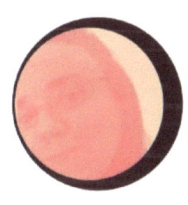

WELLCOME

WHY THIS TEXT WAS REVISED AND EXPANDED IN FEBRUARY 2020?.

I love this book very much. I published it three years ago, when I was the mother of a three-year-old boy. For two years I tried for my second pregnancy with zero success. By then, I was probably an infertile woman. 17% of Spanish women of child bearing age are, and I was one more.

Overwhelmed by my inability to have another child, I searched for 101 ways to regain my fertility when it was no longer possible. Homeopathy, "alkaline diet", estrogens and progesterones à la carte, 2 In Vitro Fertilizations failed ... Nothing worked and that nothing hurt me. Where then to draw strength for a last attempt at In Vitro Fertilization ?. Of my greatest discovery and hopefully yours too: Epigenetics.

I'm lucky. Today I have a second child: a daughter. I am the same one who wrote the book. I am infinitely grateful for the positive comments from those who have read it and the negative ones because they have helped me improve it where it was needed. This is a living being that needs maintenance. There is much to do. I finally understood. Thanks again everyone.

I love this book

Epigenetics. The DNA of the Pregnant Mother

1 EPIGENETIS. INTRODUCTION

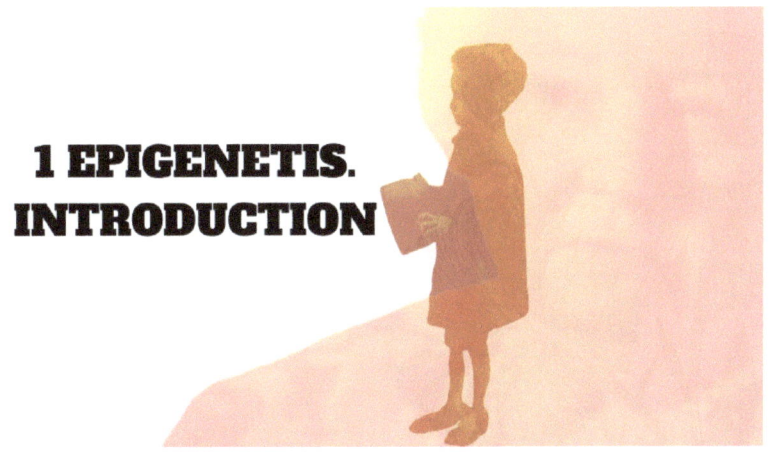

Hungry and pregnant. Holland, 1944

In 1944 pregnant women in occupied Holland only consumed 700 calories a day when they should have 2,400 calories on average.

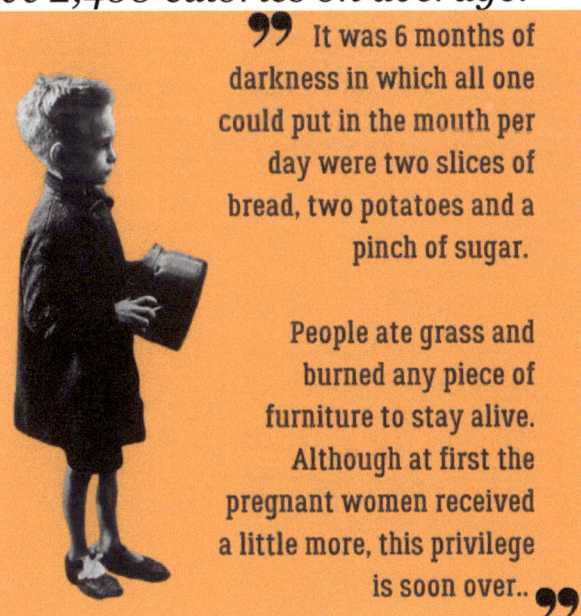

" It was 6 months of darkness in which all one could put in the mouth per day were two slices of bread, two potatoes and a pinch of sugar.

People ate grass and burned any piece of furniture to stay alive. Although at first the pregnant women received a little more, this privilege is soon over.. "

Epigenetics. The DNA of the Pregnant Mother

Loest Joost remembers how she gave birth under german occupation.

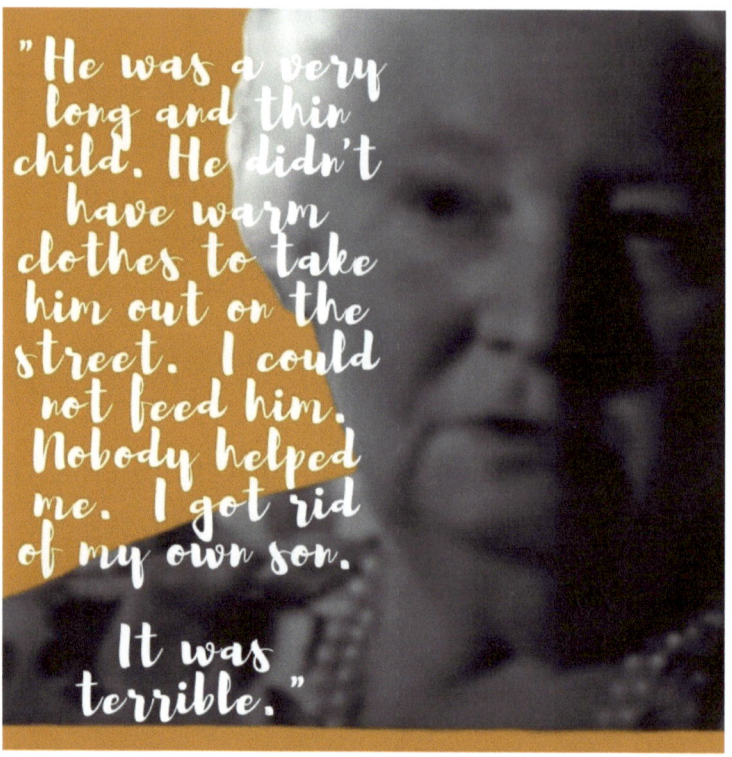

"He was a very long and thin child. He didn't have warm clothes to take him out on the street. I could not feed him. Nobody helped me. I got rid of my own son. It was terrible."

Unfortunately, children born that year suffered asthma or had a low birth weight. They used to be born short and continued to have a short stature until they reached adulthood. Although they had access to plenty of food after the war, their bodies never returned to recover from early malnutrition. They were more sensitive to stress, were more likely to suffer from coronary heart disease and their employability in the later part of their working life was surprisingly low.

The really extraordinary thing was to verify that although they had been perfectly healthy at birth, something had happened in the womb during the first months of life and that it could affect a person for the rest of his or her life as well as their offspring.

It could be said that the grandchildren and granddaughters born of these women still carried a mark without having known the hardships of war, which confirms that eggs and sperm transport the genetic adaptation of their parents and grandparents from the moment of conception.

That poor nutrition changed the genes of these war children.
 The cells have memory and acting on that memory will sooner or later produce a biological effect, store more fat and cause more heart attacks. They do not guarantee good health, but more allergies. But how can past environment cause a cardiovascular disease? Here is the explanation in a little more detail.
A malnourished baby is born expecting to stay hungry all his life. So his metabolism slows down, he

saves calories and avoids excessive exercise. The problem is that the effects of hunger are short and although living conditions can change rapidly, the methylation (changes) of DNA are slow to revert.

After hunger, abundance and plenty come to Holland after the war. However, these children have slowed metabolism: so they accumulate fat in abundance and suffer from cholesterol and type 2 diabetes. Since their body mass grows, their heart has to work harder and they develop cardiovascular diseases .

And why do survivors of the Dutch famine could also suffer more from autism, depression or schizophrenia? In addition to the fact that genetic information is written into our DNA, these genes are activated and deactivated by epigenetic switches. They are small chemical decorations called methyl-residues. When these are added to the electron-rich, amino-structures in our DNA, they can silence certain genes or activate them.

A period of famine can lead to the methylation-change of some genes that should have acted as a defense against certain diseases and not as potential dangers to your health. They are chemical transformations in DNA regions associated with environmental stress.

Epigenetics. The DNA of the Pregnant Mother

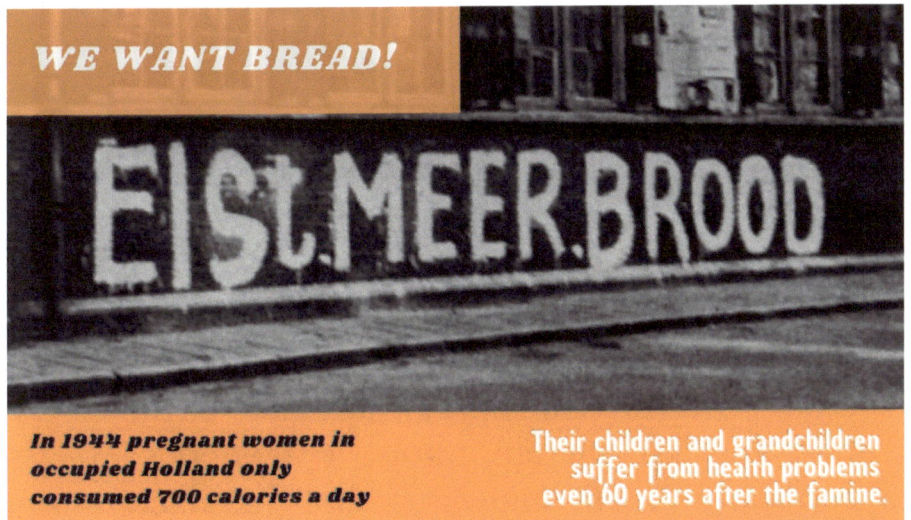

In 1944 pregnant women in occupied Holland only consumed 700 calories a day. Their children and grandchildren suffer from health problems even 60 years after the famine.

What is epigenetics?

Until after World War II it was assumed that your inheritance and personally experienced environment were the only two forces that shaped your physical appearance, your character or intelligence. Now there is a third way: epigenetics.
Epigenetics is everything that is beyond genetics. It is all apparently heritable that the DNA code and sequence fails to explain. It is beyond a standard explanation.
In 1942 the British biologist **Conrad Weddington** suggested that the correspondence between genes and traits is not simple. Biological development should be determined by many genes that affect each other and interact with the environment. He

postulated that it is possible in some way to modify your genes without altering the sequence of your DNA. In other words, that inheritance has several forms of memory: a permanent one, that is due to a change in sequence, and a more transient one, that can span few generations. The latter biological singularity will be inherited by your children and even your grandchildren.

In 1990 the British epidemiologist **David Barker** applied his knowledge about epigenetics to the mother's womb. He suggested that the placenta and the endometrium of a pregnant woman communicate with each other and that they are able to reprogram the genetics that had been given to her in an Assisted Reproduction treatment such as egg donation or surrogacy.

Epigenetics. The DNA of the Pregnant Mother

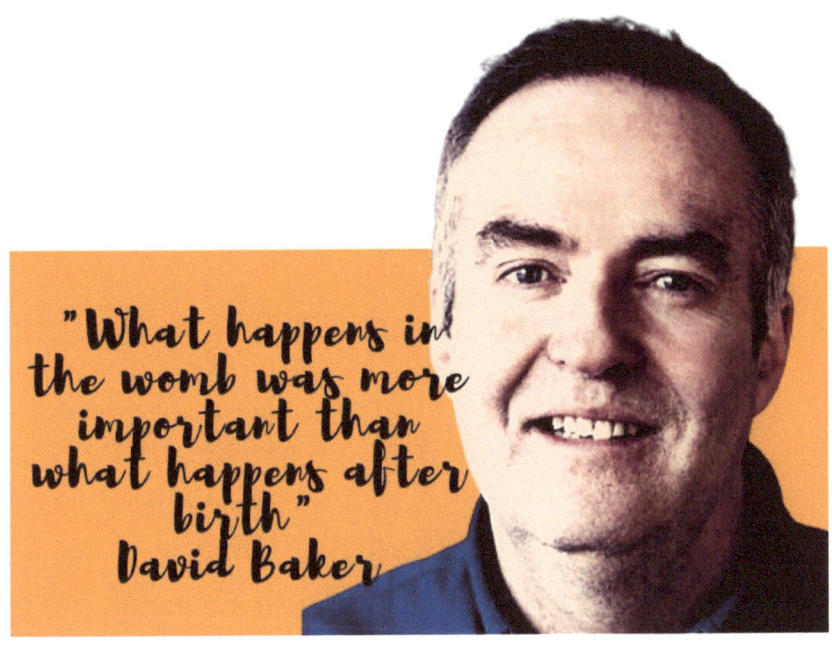

"What happens in the womb was more important than what happens after birth"
David Baker

The environment also has an influence

Genetic inheritance is not a closed treasure trove. The expression "gene on and off" means that your daily life, the experiences you live both positively and negatively, the foods you eat and the environment in which you grow have a huge influence on your genes

Many of the traumas experienced in your first years of life have consequences on your body and personality as an adult woman. Mothers who went through continued stress, violence or hunger and children who suffered abuse may suffer abnormal DNA alterations that cause them to have low tolerance for stress, autism, schizophrenia or cancer.

Remember

- Epigenetics controls the expression of genes without changing the DNA sequence itself.
- Genes are not inherited without more, your daily life, your life experiences, the food you eat and the environment in which you grow will directly influence them. This inheritance will happen to your children and even grandchildren.

Epigenetics. The DNA of the Pregnant Mother

2. WILL MY GENES SHOW UP?

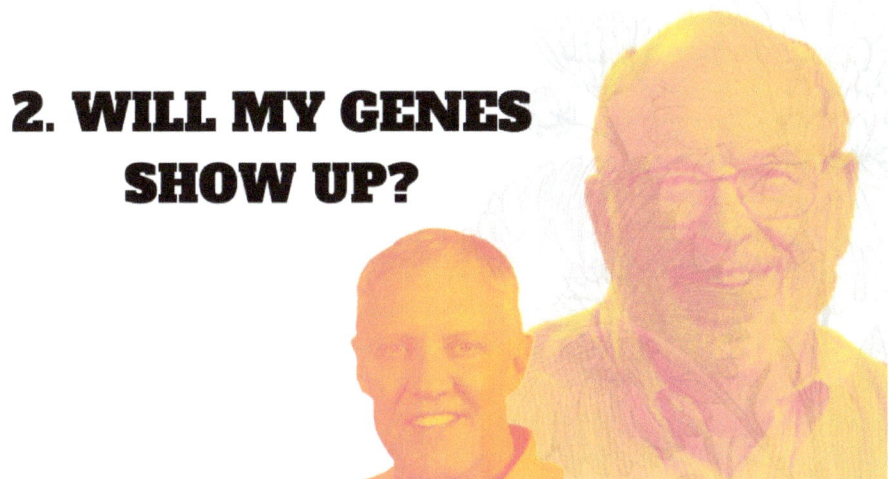

Genetic inheritance is not something completely given

*U*nlike logic or math, biology and epigenetics are empirical, "fuzzy" sciences. So you should not expect 100% to inherit a certain physical trait or the intelligence of your father or mother. You only have a higher "**probability of inheriting them**."

Physical Features

If you conceived a baby with your own ovarian egg, your baby will have a greater predisposition to inherit your physical features. However, if you needed an egg donation to fulfill your desire to be a mother, your baby will also be more likely to inherit your eyes and hair if your Donor and you both have the same or similar physical characteristics.

Intelligence (high capacities)

The same goes for intelligence, you don't inherit it by default.
It is only more likely to genetically inherit high intellectual performance, but this occurs in any social group, not just in a high social stratum.

Diseases

Another interesting side of epigenetics is that your body develops a kind of immune memory that helps defend you against infections and makes you return to a state of emotional normality after having overcome a high stress situation. Interesting, right?

Scientifically we know that epigenetic modifications help us to:

> 1. Acquire immunological memory that defends us from infections

2. Organize the cells of the nervous system that form the neurobiological base of memory
3. Return to a state of emotional normality after having overcome a situation of high stress
4. However, epigenetic mutations – EPIMUTATIONS - can also lead to psychiatric illnesses such as schizophrenia and depression, some neurological and cancer development among others.

Epimutations

Remember that your cells are sensitive to the environment in which you live.

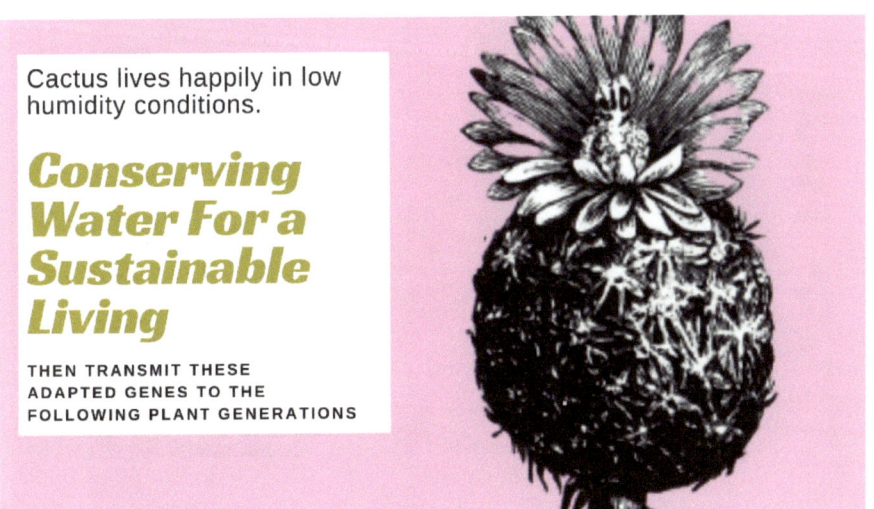

Cactus lives happily in low humidity conditions.

Conserving Water For a Sustainable Living

THEN TRANSMIT THESE ADAPTED GENES TO THE FOLLOWING PLANT GENERATIONS

Epigenetics. The DNA of the Pregnant Mother

You can develop diseases throughout your life, not just at the beginning, The good news is that they can be reversible, which opens a wide field to prevent and treat diseases of genetic origin. Scientists **Meaney y Gluckman** called this phenomenon "epimutations." Organisms adapt to the conditions in which they live.

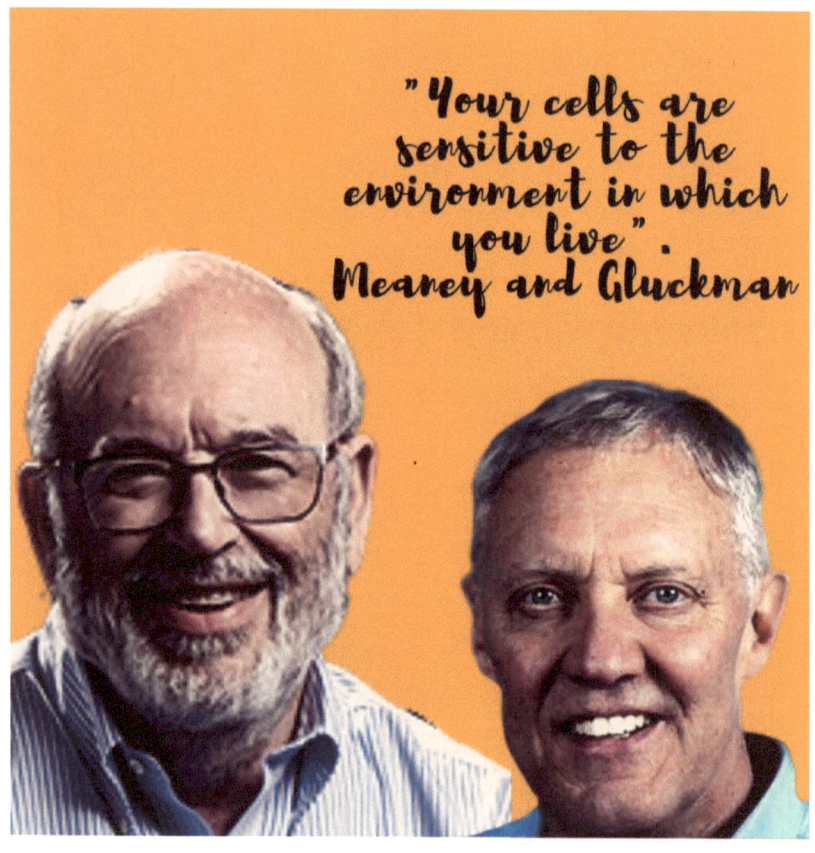

"Your cells are sensitive to the environment in which you live".
Meaney and Gluckman

Remember

- You only have the "probability of inheriting" certain physical traits or the intelligence of your parents, not a 100% certainty.
- Epigenetic modifications help you defend yourself against infections, keep your body in memory and overcome stressful situations.
- Epimutations due to environmental factors are reversible.

Epigenetics. The DNA of the Pregnant Mother

3. DETRIMENTAL EPIGENETIC MEMORY

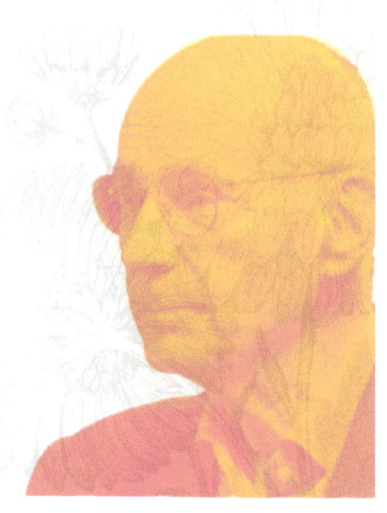

Genetic sensitivity

We already know that your cells are able to remember "the environment that surrounds them", and cause a stable change in your body or behavior without altering the sequence of your DNA.

The genetics of your baby is more easily marked if you lived in a hostile environment at the time of conception, being an embryo, in your childhood and puberty.

Epigenetics. The DNA of the Pregnant Mother

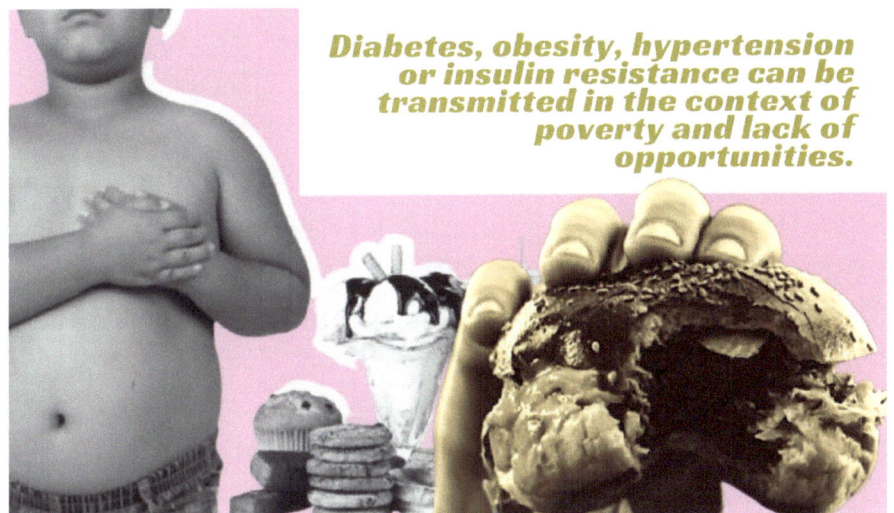

Diabetes, obesity, hypertension or insulin resistance can be transmitted in the context of poverty and lack of opportunities.

We review some of the factors that negatively influence your baby from the embryonic phase to the end of his adult stage.

A) About embryo

An inhospitable environment does not favor any pregnancy. Modifying cells, proteins and nucleic acids of Your endometrium, could alter Your baby's genetics. For example by adding or removing certain chemical compounds in its DNA (methylation or demethylation), which could predispose later to mental illnesses such as autism, depression or schizophrenia.

1. **High levels of stress or violence:** high levels of anxiety hormone (adrenaline, corticosterone) or the presence of hormones antagonizing blood insulin (glucagone, glucocorticosteroids) cause your baby to grow less, and predispose to high blood pressure and coronary heart disease, glucose intolerance, anxiety disorders, depression or schizophrenia.

2. **Malnutrition of the mother:** the growth of your baby is slower, its intellectual progress could also be delayed, in addition to causing permanent changes in his brain or developing chronic diseases.

3. **Exposure to tobacco (smoking or vaping):** Since nicotine is vasoconstrictive, it reduces the flow of maternal blood containing nutrients to the baby ("chemical starvation"). Smoke carbon monoxide also decreases blood oxygen transport, producing partial "chemical strangulation". In addition, active or passive smoking increases your own risk of cancer.

4. **Drinking alcohol:** In addition to being a cell toxin, alcohol also opens ligand-dependent chloride channels in the brain. Under exposure to alcohol the baby grows less, and may show facial

irregularities, become hyperactive and develop cognitive deficits and memory disorder.

B) Chilhood and puberty

We know that the problems suffered in childhood can translate into health disorders in adulthood, a child with problems is an adult prone to cancer.

Lack of attachment figure: the absence of a stable adult in the life of a minor, whether due to illness, deprivation of liberty, violence or distance, causes an increase in chronic endocrine and mental illnesses in response to a hostile environment.

Boris Cyrulnik, French holocaust survivor, double orphan, neuropsychiatrist, psychoanalyst, coined the term "resilience", as a predisposition and a way to rebuild a life after having experienced a trauma.

Epigenetics. The DNA of the Pregnant Mother

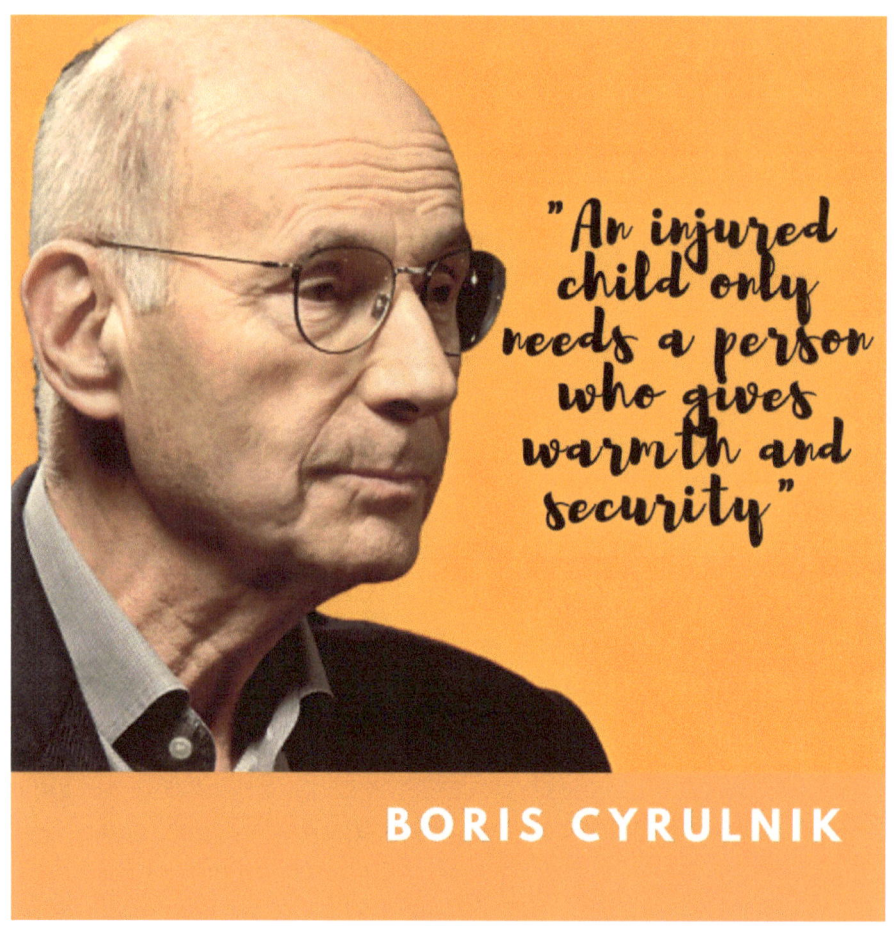

Emotional state of caregivers: if the mother suffers from depression or stress, you should know that this also directly affects the emotional development of her children.

Father or mother who are not involved in raising their children or giving them affection maintain "an avoidance attachment," which is associated with a reduced ability to learn and memorize.

Poverty is hereditory: if there are less economic resources, there are also less educational and employment opportunities. This is the perfect environment to perpetuate poverty from generation to generation by simple inertia.

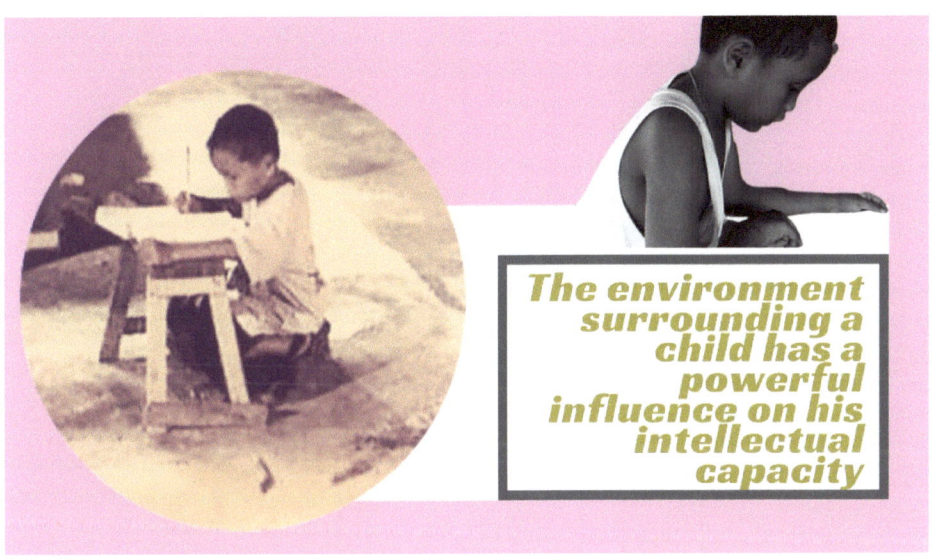

The environment surrounding a child has a powerful influence on his intellectual capacity

Remember

• The exposure of the mother during pregnancy to situations of stress, violence, malnutrition, tobacco smoking and alcohol causes stunted embryo growth, less intellectual progress, chronic diseases, increased risk of cancer, hyperactivity, facial

irregularities, cognitive deficits and memory mismatches.
- Other environmental factors that negatively condition genes until they reach adulthood are the lack of a figure of secure attachment, parents / caregivers' depression or stress disorder, as well as the lack of financial resources.

Epigenetics. The DNA of the Pregnant Mother

4. GENES FOR HEALTH

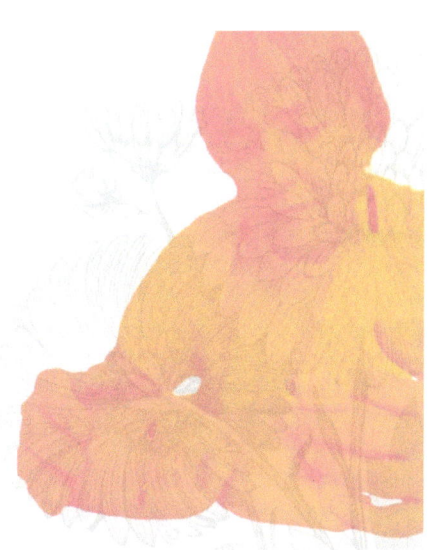

From Health Genes to Illness Genes

The genes you inherit shape your physical appearance and decide whether you are sick or not, but you are not a prisoner of your genes, nor can you hide in them. We are not predetermined irreversibly by genes. This is what **Craig Venter**, a biologist specializing in human genome, strongly indicates:

Epigenetics. The DNA of the Pregnant Mother

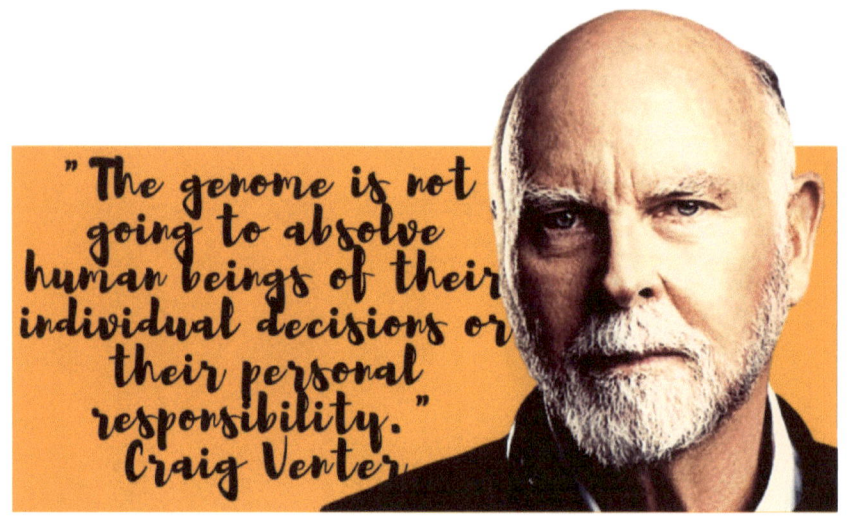

"The genome is not going to absolve human beings of their individual decisions or their personal responsibility."
Craig Venter

"No can take refuge behind their genes"

Your behavior is determined in part by the genes you inherit and by your personal and social circumstances in two opposite directions:
1. activating health genes and silencing disease genes or vice versa

2. mutating healthy genes into disease genes

Epigenetics. The DNA of the Pregnant Mother

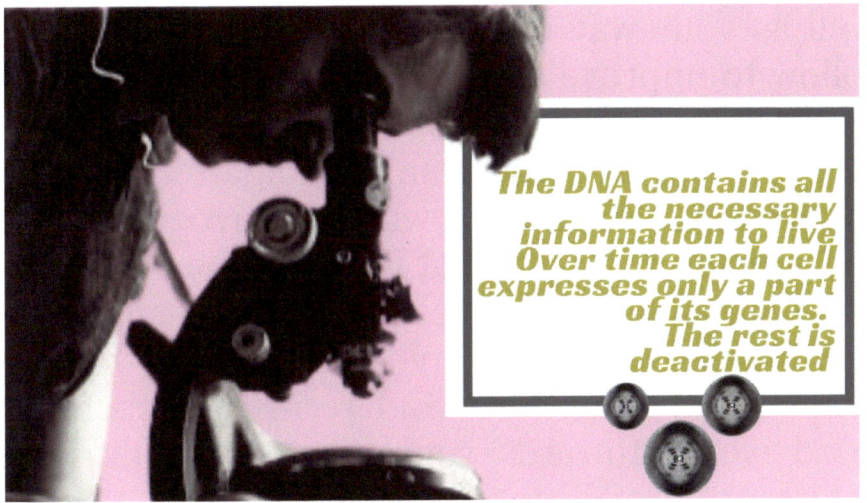

The DNA contains all the necessary information to live. Over time each cell expresses only a part of its genes. The rest is deactivated

Nutrition and maternal womb

The pregnant woman who consumes less than 2,400 calories of quality a day exposes her baby to lower growth and chronic diseases such as obesity, diabetes, and cardiovascular problems in adulthood.

10 daily routines that reformat your baby's DNA inside your uterus

10 daily routines that reformat your baby's DNA inside your uterus
Your baby is the reflection of your genetic load, that of your partner and that of your grandparents, as

well as your way of life, but what strategy can you follow to improve the genetic footprint you leave on your offspring from the moment of that you conceive them? How can a woman receiving an ovarian egg donation or who's a surrogate reformat the genetics of an egg that is not her own?. There are at least 10 daily routines available to all pregnant women. It does not require money, but huge amounts of time, love, and recurring repetition of good works towards your new tenant during the nine months of gestation:

> 1. **Touch:** is the first sense to develop, you are designed to need physical contact from birth to the end of your days. This sensitivity helps the baby without vision in the uterus to send stimuli to his senses and nervous system.
>
> According to psychologist **Tiffany Field** of the Touch Research Institute in Miami:

Epigenetics. The DNA of the Pregnant Mother

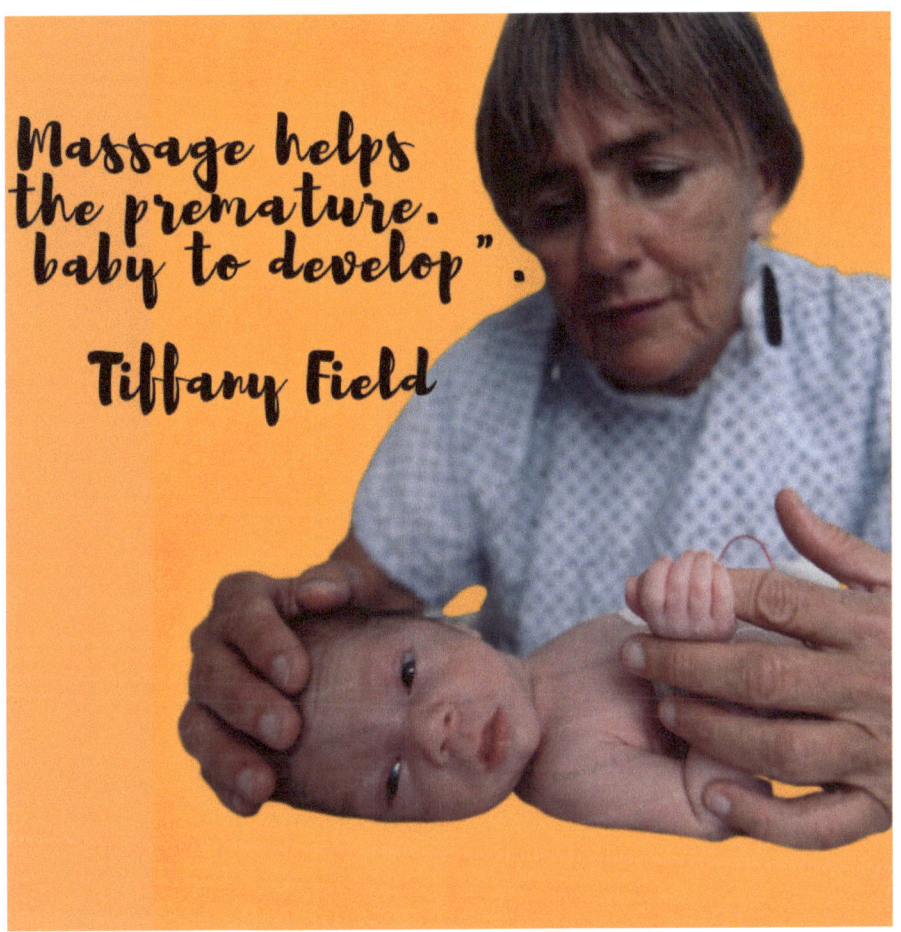

"Massage helps the premature baby to develop". Tiffany Field

"When someone is hugged with love, the pressure receptors under the skin that send a sensation to the spinal cord and brainstem are stimulated, which reduces the heart rate and stress hormones (cortisol), facilitates the digestion and absorption of food, besides reducing pain"

Caress your baby belly frequently, because the baby will develop much better in life and will be less predisposed to suffer from asthma, autism, diabetes, dermatitis, autoimmune diseases, depression or attention disorders

2. Healthy nutrition and intellectual performance:

A poor diet of the mother during pregnancy can cause permanent changes in the structure and functioning of her baby's brain.

The brain is built by the proteins, lipids, carbohydrates, vitamins and minerals that you eat from food; It is the most metabolically active organ. Because of having very limited energy reserves, you need to continually stock up on glucose.

3. Positive experiences: they make you feel good. They open your mind, recharge you with energy, and provide an emotional cushion to deal with traumatic or stressful situations such as pregnancy, they make you recover from adversity. They reduce the levels of the stress hormone 'cortisol', and even the physical pain that causes stress.

4. Reduce chronic stress or fear: it decreases your ability to digest food,

- ignores the function of insulin: by increasing your appetite, you burn less fat, and you favor the transmission of obesity and diabetes
- inhibits the production of NK cells that destroy cancer cells and viruses
- accelerates the growth of cancer cells
- your baby grows less

5. Plays and games: The information stored in the brain is transmitted through dendrites, which are extensions of neuronal cells similar to the branches of a tree. Neurons will extend their branches or create new ones with games that improve memory, concentration, attention, response time, verbal and nonverbal reasoning... Simply playing to tie your shoes or brushing your teeth with the opposite hand will stimulate one or two neurons.

Prenatal and postnatal stimulation will help your baby to:
- pay attention for longer periods, learn faster and be more curious
  - develop greater neuronal density, improve memory, auditory and linguistic intelligence, sense of touch, visual, balance, or dexterity
  - improve blood circulation to the brain

Most of the information stored in the brain actually resides in extensions of cells resembling the branches of a tree called **dendrites**. We can extend their branches or create new ones with games that improve memory, concentration, attention, response time, verbal and non-verbal reasoning, etc. Simply playing tying your shoes or brushing your teeth with the opposite hand, It will stimulate one or two neurons.

6. **Positive attitude**: a pregnancy is a natural process that needs to change your sleep pattern, your diet, your digestion, your breathing, your smell, your taste, your eyesight and even your touch...

Consultations to the gynecologist, maternity classes, prenatal gymnastics, midwife visits...

try to do away your fear as a first-time mother. Give yourself security and support within a group of women equal to you. In addition to preventing possible physical disorders such as gestational diabetes or sciatica, this will improve your emotional status! It's about living your pregnancy with the best predisposition so that:

- endorphins and neurotransmitters help you maintain a more vital mood
- strengthen your immune system
- have a faster physical and emotional recovery after delivery
- you can be more resistant, yield less to stress or depression during pregnancy or postpartum. And if you give in, try not to wallow in a paralyzing frustration.

> *"A positive attitude begins with a healthy self-image. If you like the way you are and you are satisfied, confident and sure of yourself, others will feel the same about you"*

- being more resistant, giving less to stress or depression during gestation or postpartum. And if you do give in, to not suffer from paralyzing frustration.

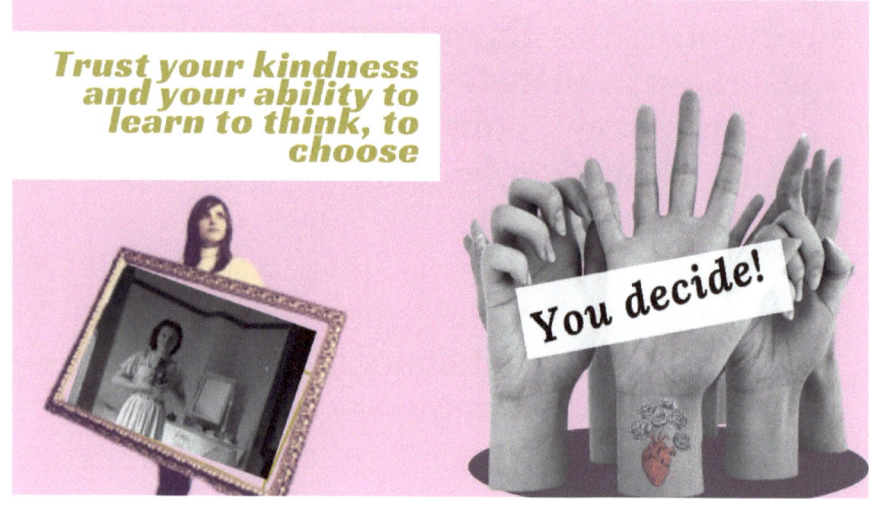

7. Moderate physical exercise: moderate and supervised physical activity during your pregnancy favors so much to the baby,
 • its brain is more mature weeks after birth
 • its heart rate is more marked
 • the baby forms new neurons, new neurotransmitters and other brain growth factors, facilitates memory, learning, concentration, and alertness

like you,

- the exercise also helps you better overcome some of the typical discomforts of pregnancy such as low back pain or sciatica
- relieves fluid retention or swelling of legs
- improves your elasticity when you delay in childbirth
- releases accumulated tension, reduces stress, depression, irritability or bad mood
- stimulates the release of endorphins, distracts from worries, has fun and facilitates a healthy lifestyle

One should also mention also for biology researchers **Juleen Zierath and Romain Barres** of the Karolinska Institute in Stockholm (Sweden), who demonstrated how physical exercise could inhibit the onset of diabetes, thanks to a biochemical process known as methylation / demethylation (activation or deactivation) of genes.

Epigenetics. The DNA of the Pregnant Mother

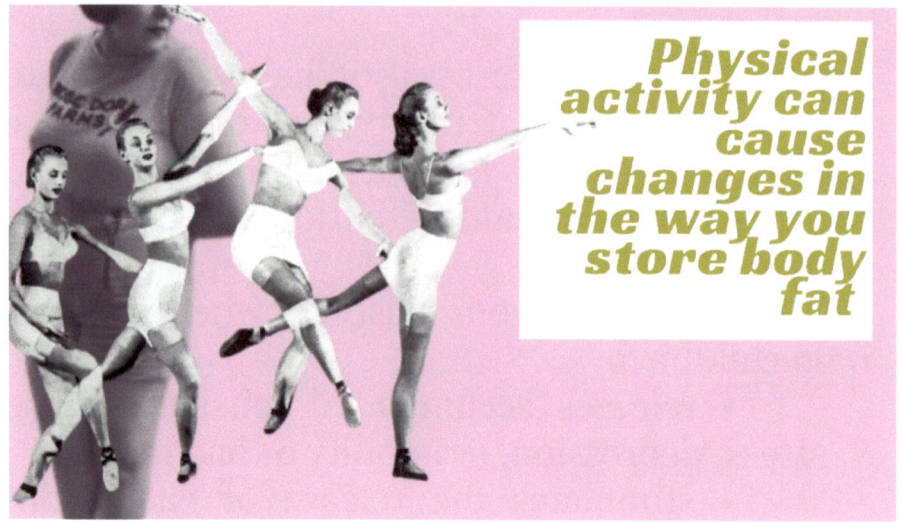

Babies born with excessive accumulated fat as a result of the mother's high blood sugar levels during pregnancy (gestational diabetes) tend to stay obese during childhood and adulthood. These babies are also predisposed to **hipoglucemia** (low blood sugar levels) during childhood and adolescence due to an epigenetic effect of high insulin production.

8. **Safe attachment:** Thanks to the love and dedication of those who cared for us in our childhood, the brain of an adult will have good neurotransmitters prepared to face the challenges of life with more or less joy and to return affection.

Epigenetics. The DNA of the Pregnant Mother

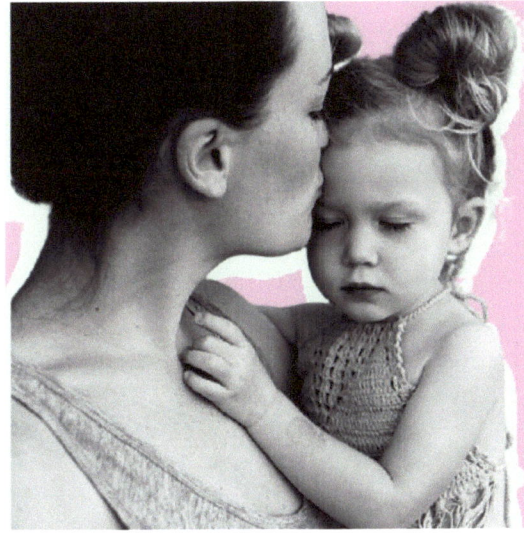

Healthy and safe childhood attachment builds your future adult emotional stability and develops your resources to overcome difficult situations

The key to creating resilient adults is a healthy and safe childhood attachment during childhood. So that at some point in your life you have had in your environment an example of what a protective figure should be.

<u>Thomas R. Verny</u>, a psychiatrist and an authority in the study of the influence of the environment on the baby before and after birth states that:

> *"During the first two years of life the maturation of the brain is linked with that of your caregiver to produce the right hormones and neurotransmitters in the correct sequence. This tuning determines the permanent cerebral architecture "*

Epigenetics. The DNA of the Pregnant Mother

According to **Siegel**, a psychiatrist and biologist at the University of California, affection between the child and the caregiver is more important than sensory stimulation:

> *"Parents do not need to stimulate their children excessively. Instead of bombarding them with sensation cues, what they need to be able to grow properly is to be with their caregivers."*

Although the brain remains malleable until adulthood, we know that most of its connections form in the first 3 years of life. Your baby needs a secure attachment with its caregivers, whether it's you, your parents or other guardians, so that it will feel accepted and confident, that is when it will be curious to discover their surroundings, to learn with others.

The quality of attachment will also influence the development of empathy, the modulation of desires and impulses, the feeling of belonging and the ability to give and receive.

9. **Voice and language:** talk to your baby when he or she is inside your belly, in this way you favor its neuronal and emotional development. In addition you strengthen the emotional bonds between you two.

Your baby will start listening to you from the 24th week of gestation. Your vocal cords vibrate and that vibration travels through your bones to your pelvic cavity

- during the first phase of pregnancy, your baby begins to play with his or her body to the rhythm of your voice
- In the last weeks, eliminate your baby's stress and anxiety due to its large size and the pressure of the uterine arteries, which make it difficult for oxygen to enter its brain
- and when he or she is born, hearing your voice calms the baby

If during these times you do not know what to say, just tell the baby how you are that day, what plans you have. Tell the baby at all times that you love it very much.

The researchers from the University of Kansas (USA), **Betty Hart y Todd Risley**, highlight the influence of communication on the high intellectual abilities (intelligence) of children:

• high intellectual performance (intelligence) and the ability to communicate is related to the number of words parents speak to their daughters or sons
• the academic success of children at ages 9 and 10 is connected to the number of words they heard from birth to three years of age

10. **Give food:** it is a very powerful demonstration of affection. Giving food is speaking to the most primitive form of the brain, it is like telling a baby it is cared for and protected. Transmit your love and your ability to care for the baby. So when it feels distressed, dissatisfied or unloved, it is more tempted to turn to food.

However, beware of being overweight, especially during pregnancy.

Reproductive health

What to you eat and how much it could improve your fertility.

Before you get pregnant it is advisable to clean your body of toxins to create an optimal environment in which the embryo can develop healthily, in addition to improving your health and well-being.

A) Nutrients

Nutrients are chemicals that make up food. The organism uses them for its development, activity and maintenance. They also provide energy to the body.

1. **Mineral Zinc and vitamin B6:** affect all parts of the female sexual cycle, relieve pre-menstrual problems.

• Zinc is found in nuts, egg yolks, rye, green leafy vegetables, sunflower seeds, fish and bran.
• B6 is found in cauliflower, canon, bananas and broccoli.

2. **Omega-3 and -6 fatty acids**: they are needed for cell membrane fluidity and as raw materials for essential tissue hormones (postaglandins, prostacyclines).
Eat a serving of fatty fish such as mackerel, sardines and salmon two or three times a week and eat a tablespoon of raw seeds without salt every day.

3. **Vitamin C and E:** Antioxidants

- Vitamin C is found in green leafy vegetables, peppers, kiwis, tomatoes, citrus fruits and blueberries
- Vitamin E is in nuts, pipes, fatty fish, avocados, beans and sweet potatoes

4. **Vitamin A (vegetable beta-carotene):** it is necessary for the growth of the ovarian eggs prior to ovulation.
It is found in carrots, sweet potatoes, dried apricots, fruit juices and watercress

5. **Selenium:** Is present in Brazil nuts, sesame seeds, tuna, cabbage and whole wheat flour.

B) Antinutrients

They make no nutritional contribution to your body and deplete your vital resources, which reduces fertility.

1. Sugar: Robs large amounts of vitamins and minerals from the body for its own processing.

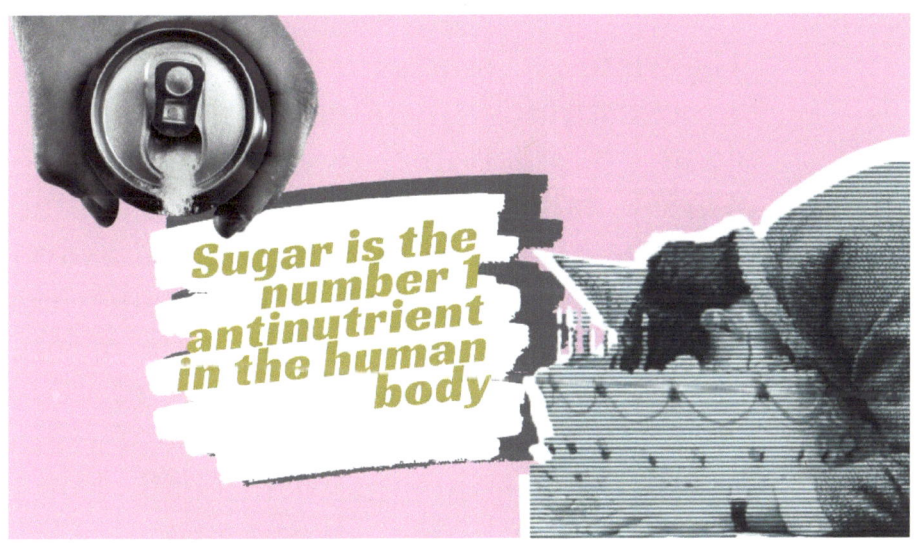

Sugar is the number 1 antinutrient in the human body

1. **Alcohol:** not only does it have toxic effects on the male reproductive system. In addition to producing a significant deterioration in sperm quality, it can cause physical, behavioral and mental

development abnormalities during fetal development

2. Tobacco: Cigarette smoke impairs the quality of your ovaries and their DNA – their survival code - and has serious consequences on mental and physical development. Maternal smoking increases the risk of having a premature baby or having a miscarriage.

Cigarette smoke contains the vasoconstrictor nicotine which impairs blood circulation to inner organs – ovaries, fallopian tubes and the womb, reducing overall egg quality as well as that of its DNA, our survival code, which has far more serious consequences on mental and physical development of the baby. Smoking downgrades female fertility making conception more difficult, but it also speeds up aging, bringing menopause forward. Even when a baby is conceived, smoking reduces blood supply to the baby – a chemical famine – and thus increases the risk of having a premature baby or having an abortion.

3. Endocrine-Disruptor Chemicals: These chemicals can unbalance your sexual hormone levels and cause birth defects, as well as cognitive and neurodevelopmental abnormalities in your baby. They are found in paint, plastics, food product containers, pesticides, cosmetics, perfumes, etc. Workers of the textile industry, nurses who handle drugs against cancer and all those who usually work with dyes, solvents and herbicides are exposed to them in a greater extent

Sexually transmitted diseases and bacterial infections: reduce fertility and increase the risk of abortion.

7. **Stress:** consumes resources of essential nutrients for reproduction, especially vitamin B and inhibits ovulation of women.

The contraceptive pill: Consumes essential nutrients such as vitamin B and C, and also increases the level of copper – for some time after being discontinued - causing later subfertility and birth defects. Stop using it at least three months before trying to conceive so that you recover your normal menstrual cycle.

8. **Toxic metals:** Lead and mercury from poor quality paints or old dental fillings can influence your fertility and harm the fetus.

9. **Homocystein:** is a modified amino-acid that is found naturally in our blood. High levels of homocystein are associated with a diet lacking in nutrients or can be due to a genetic problem can result in infertility.

10. **Dairy**: too much milk, yogurt or cheese are foods that can cause acidity in both the stomach and your vagina, creating an environment that is not conducive for sperm to survive in your cervix

Remember

• Your behavior is the result of your genetic inheritance, your personal and social circumstances. Activate your health genes and silence those of disease or vice versa.

Epigenetics. The DNA of the Pregnant Mother

- There are at least 10 routines that reformat your baby's DNA from the mother's womb such as physical contact, healthy naturition, play, absence of stress or fear, physical exercise, secure attachment or mother's voice
- Consume quality nutrients to improve your fertility

5. EPIGENETICS IN ASSISTED REPRODUCTION

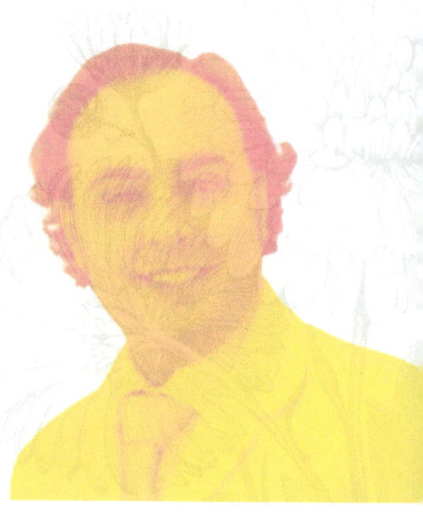

Road start (Kilometer 0): I am infertile.

*H*aving children is one of the most exciting life projects a woman can have. We are biologically programmed to give life. We assume that we can procreate by nature, but something fails when the years pass and the desired pregnancy does not arrive.

We need courage to recognize that we are no longer so fertile. We need help to be mothers. Having a son or daughter becomes a unique goal. Each failed attempt, each new menstruation adds anxiety and the bank account decreases.

We are women who at some point have felt the burden that our body is not able to achieve a spontaneous pregnancy. Or that we regret having delayed motherhood for too long: the scholarly women's curse.

If we accept the fact that we do not have in our hands the supreme power to create life, we are in a position to overcome a barrier, that of not having our dream children. Now it's time to find them in an alternative way. It is necessary to be flexible.

Active reception of ovarian eggs. You are not a passive mom

Accepting the genes of another anonymous woman to fulfill the dream of being a mother is not a simple decision. First you have to accept infertility in the first person and then overcome the initial rejection of egg donation. Unfortunately, hospitals and fertility clinics project the discouraging image of pregnant women as a merely passive recipient of ovarian eggs or embryos.

Epigenetics. The DNA of the Pregnant Mother

However, **epigenetics recently demonstrated that the woman who carries an embryo not genetically related to her can nevertheless influence it**, facilitating the expression of some genes and silencing that of others. Thus she is reformatting the genetic code she receives till she gives birth. To a baby. You are not a mere passive receiver.

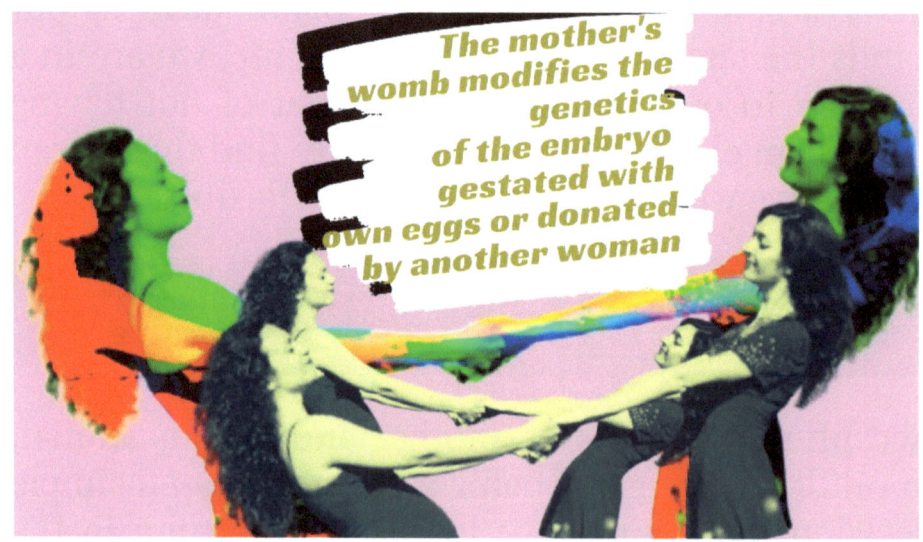

The mother's womb modifies the genetics of the embryo gestated with own eggs or donated by another woman

For the baby, its mother's womb carries and contributes more than the donor woman because we are a union of inherited genes and a way of life. Our day to day, our diet, the medications we take, cigarettes, alcohol, drugs... everything has its epigenetic counterpart, until we live our pregnancies with joy.

Epigenetics. The DNA of the Pregnant Mother

The pregnant mother does contribute. Exchange between endometrium and embryo

When a woman becomes pregnant at her home, without going through the roller of hospitals and fertility clinics, what she transmits to her baby is a half of her genetic load and the whole regulation of the DNA. But in the case of a baby born by egg donation, embryo donation or surrogacy, can it have a piece of its pregnant mother or will it be an "alien" in her womb?

A woman with or without a partner, a female couple or a woman who lends her womb as a surrogate – these women who have already assumed that they need the help of another woman to become a mother, are surely interested in knowing the results from the Valencian Institute of Infertility Foundation (FIVI) on its 2 year-long investigation on the effects of embryo modification.

<u>Felipe Vilella</u>, researcher at the Foundation of the Instituto Valenciano de la Infertilidad (FIVI, Valencia, Spain), and **Carlos Simón** (Stanford University, Ca, US) demonstrated the existence of

communication between the pregnant mother and her embryo in a study entitled '**HSA-miR-30d secreted by the human endometrium, is taken up by the pre-implantation embryo and might modify its** transcriptome' published in the high-impact journal Development in 2015.

The study explores the communication between the endometrium and the embryo just before implantation, identifying a specific molecule of the endometrial fluid (hsa-miR-30d) that is able to reprogram embryonic genetics by modifying the expression of genes, which makes specific functions expressed or inhibited in this embryo.

With this pioneering work, the authors confirmed the Barker hypothesis, first formulated by English epidemiologist David Barker in 1990 that states that what happens in the womb is more important than what happens after birth.

As Felipe Vilella explains:

Epigenetics. The DNA of the Pregnant Mother

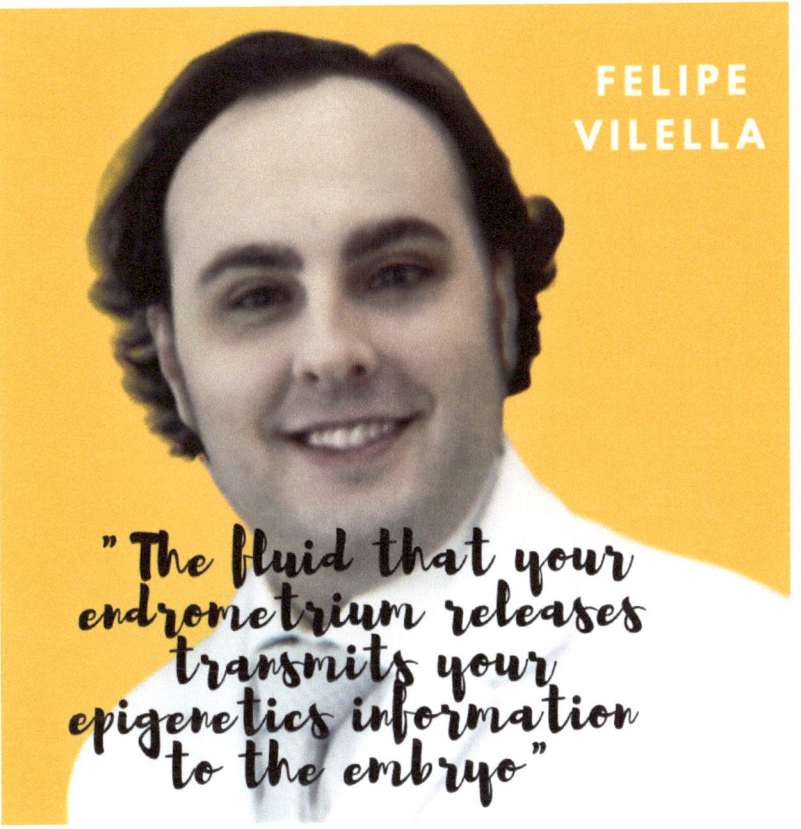

FELIPE VILELLA

"The fluid that your endometrium releases transmits your epigenetics information to the embryo"

"Although the pregnant mother does not transmit a copy of her whole genetic load to the embryo (at best, it is just 50%), she can modify all of it. It applies even if the ovarian egg was from a donor, which completely changes the paradigm of egg donation and uterus surrogation.

Epigenetics. The DNA of the Pregnant Mother

> *This opens the door of hope for those mothers who have to resort to oocyte donation to fulfill their reproductive desires and alerts those who opt for a uterus surrogacy to the pathologies that replacement mothers can transmit during pregnancy. Such as obesity, smoking, schizophrenia or diabetes."*

A possibility of transmitting physical features or cognitive and character traits of the pregnant mother to the next generation?

Felipe Vilella believes that it is like this:

> *"If it is known that there are certain diseases that have an epigenetic origin, then certain physical traits of children born by donating gametes with the pregnant mother could have the same origin. Genetically it is not yours, but you are giving it something from you!"*

Epigenetics. The DNA of the Pregnant Mother

The fluid that your endometrium releases transmits epigenetic information from the pregnant woman to the embryo, thus modifying its development. There is therefore a communication between endometrium and embryo. Some physical traits can coincide between mothers and children by donation of eggs / embryos.

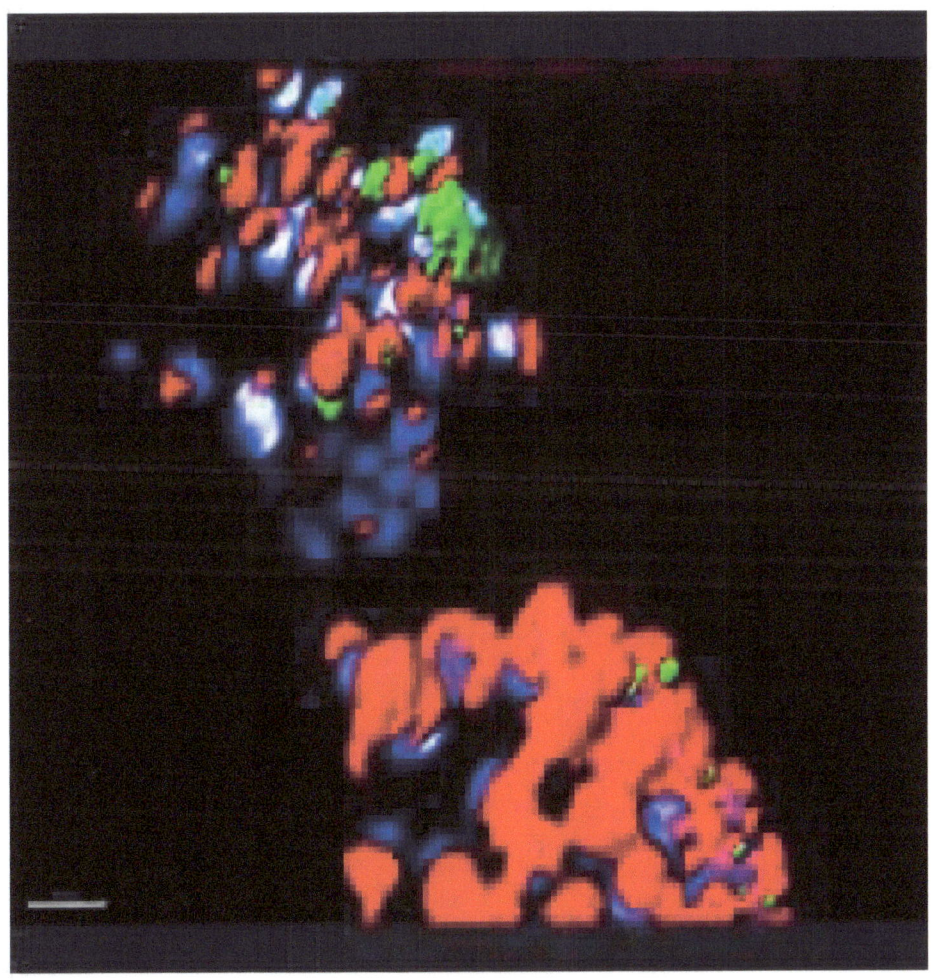

Epigenetics. The DNA of the Pregnant Mother

*Video: **The mother can modify the genetics of her son even if it is not biologically hers**"*
Source: Antena 3 TV.

The image shows in blue (gray in a black and white image) the nuclei: this is where the embryonic DNA from the woman who donated the ovarian egg is located. The microRNAs that comes from the pregnant mother and enters the embryonic cells is shown in red (white in a black and white image).

The researcher of the Valencian Institute of Infertility (IVI) Felipe Vilella describes the sequence of DNA modification produced by the pregnant mother:

> *"After the merger of egg and sperm, the newly created embryo leaves the fallopian tubes and reaches the uterus in 24 or 36 hours. It then adheres to the endometrium. During that time the pregnant mother secretes endometrial fluid that carries epigenetic information (microRNAs) which is absorbed by the embryo. The goal is to tell the embryo that everything is ready to continue the process of nesting (implantation) and development "*

Epigenetics. The DNA of the Pregnant Mother

<u>Natalia Fernández Piri</u>, coordinator of the Department of Genetics IVI Buenos Aires comments on the interaction of the endometrial RNA from the pregnant woman and embryonic DNA:

> "The micro RNA (micro-ribonucleic acid) molecules are packaged in many small 'sacs' called 'exosomes' which come in direct contact with the embryo, there taken through its surface and ferried to the cellular nuclei which Is where embryonic DNA (dysoxidoribonucleic acid) sits.
> This molecular communication the pregnant mother to be and embryonic DNA - is going to regulate the expression of some genes and not others, modifying the genetic code of the embryo before the implantation".

Epigenetics. The DNA of the Pregnant Mother

> *"Micro-RNA molecules (small ribonucleic acids) navigate in a kind of 'sachets' called 'exosomes' through the endometrial fluid and come in direct contact with the embryonic nuclei, which is where the DNA (disoxydibonucleic acid) is.*
>
> *This communication between endometrial molecules from the pregnant mother and the DNA of the embryo - whose ovum came from another woman - will switch on some genes and switch off others, modifying the genetic code of the embryo before nesting (nidation, implantation)".*

The released endometrial fluid will carry epigenetic information from the pregnant woman that will be taken by the embryo and modify its development.

Felipe Vilella highlights the importance of the information released by the endometrial fluid as follows:

Epigenetics. The DNA of the Pregnant Mother

> *"Knowing that this transmission exists, it will be possible to end the linkage of mothers to obese children. In cases of uterus surrogacy, it will also give more importance to the history of previous habits of the pregnant surrogate."*

The image shows in **blue** (*gray in a black and white image*) the nuclei where the DNA of the embryo coming from the **egg donor** woman is placed. And in **red** (*white in a black and white image*) microRNAs that come from the **pregnant mother** and enter the cells of the embryo.

The researcher of the Valencian Institute of Infertility (IVI) Felipe Vilella describes the sequence of the modification of the DNA received by the pregnant mother:

Epigenetics. The DNA of the Pregnant Mother

> "After the fertilization of ovum and spermatozoon, the embryo leaves the fallopian tubes and reaches the uterus in 24 to 36 hours, then adheres to the endometrium. Once the embryo is in the uterus, the pregnant mother to be secretes endometrial fluid with chemicals containing genetic information (microRNAs) which is absorbed by the embryo. "The goal is to tell you that everything is ready to continue the process of implantation and development."

The released small RNAs in the endometrial fluid provide genetic information from the pregnant woman to be, that is taken by the embryo, modifying its development.

Felipe Vilella reveals the importance of the information released by miRNAs in the endometrial fluid:

> "Knowing that this transmission exists, you can detect how to cut it by ending the chain of mothers with obese children, In cases of uterine surrogacy, by giving more importance to the history of previous habits of the pregnant mother"

Similar and not by chance

The environment around the baby influences it from the moment it is conceived until the end of its days. You have the opportunity to leave your mark on other people.

Mothers and fathers can stimulate the baby's brain even in the womb. Once the baby is born, its family, friends, teachers / tutors can participate in the development of its abilities, listening to its first words, showing their affection or valuing each and every of its small achievements.

Up to three years of age, the little ones need to go on their arms, and up to ten they will continue to be totally dependent beings who need at least one adult who is present 'here and now'. To take care of them with dedication, who feels like playing together, to help them with the school chores of the school or to watch together the TV performances. To ask them why they are sad or why 'the navel hurts' and that they help them to look for the toys that they have lost, showing them affection day by day, teaching them to have respect, to overcome small challenges, to calm down.

May they hear a 'love you' by surprise.

The way in which the adult behaves with the minor is related to his or her own personality. If a person is affectionate, it probably will be same with his or her own son or daughter.

These children will show same gestures as mom, dad's smile and they will be glued to the grandmother thanks to the fact that the pregnant mother 'reprogrammed' the genetic load of an egg or embryo donation during pregnancy, and for having raised her from her womb.

The personality of the children does not depend on egg donation

The infertile woman is arrested in a state of frustration at not being able to be a mother naturally. Being fertile is something that is desired but that has not been given.

If you believe that your son or daughter's personality depends strictly on genes, when a problem appears, you will think that you are not responsible for their actions. Instead, you may blame the genes introduced by the donated egg.

Non-genetic biological fathers and mothers should know that they leave their epigenetic imprint on their children, which is no small matter. During pregnancy and upbringing that lasts many years, they will modify the genes of their sons or daughters for better or worse, since what really coalesces a family is the friction and love of each day.

To tell or to keep quiet in the larger family

Under normal circumstances, you shouldn't hide that you needed the generosity of another woman to create life. Particularly, when it is only strictly revealed for medical reasons and at the moment when you know that your son or daughter is prepared to know their complete genetic identity.

If you experienced it as a difficult period with a happy ending, your offspring will probably also accept it. Or maybe not. That may depend on their criteria.

You can also find the maternal side of child's family will refuse to consider this child as 'of the same blood'. In this case, the parents can continue with their life project without being obliged to reveal the genetic origin of their children to those who they do not consider it appropriate. They can share the genetic information of their children with all their surroundings. Or with anyone. Or with the most receptive. Or only with their doctor. Your silence belongs to you, but you are slave to each of your uttered words.

Anonymous vs known donor?

If you opt for egg or embryo donation in Spain, you will not be able to know who your female donor is. By law only public hospitals and private fertility clinics have the privilege of being able to know the physical traits and clinical history of your donor(s).

However, contact with them may be established if a judge orders this in case of serious illness of the minor. For example, if a child has leukemia and requires a bone marrow transplant from a genetically closely related person.

Personally, I think it would not hurt that Spanish law in Assisted Reproduction allowed anonymous and non-anonymous donors to co-exist at the same time (even if these were the least). An adult born due to an egg or embryo donation should be able to get to know their complete genetic identity if they so wish. Because while the donors are anonymous people, without their genetic contribution, he / she would not exist.

Do Assisted Reproduction Techniques (ART) leave an epigenetic mark?

Beckwith-Wiedemann syndrome produces intrauterine overgrowth, chromosomal abnormalities, risk of childhood tumors, etc.. The **Angelman**'s syndrom causes severe intellectual retardation, poor motor coordination, excitability, and other symptoms. Both syndromes are classical imprinting disorders, ie they are known to be caused by abnormalities in epigenetic programming during embryo development.

Over the last 15years, it has been shown that there is 3 to 6 times the risk of these syndroms occurring in children born by in vitro treatments. Even though these syndroms are rare, even with ART (1:1000 or less), this is a risk that must be known and consented to, in cases of egg or embryo donation.

In general, assisted reproduction techniques such as in vitro fertilization (IVF) and ICSI (intra-cytoplasmic sperm injection) can in rare cases leave a mark. But in most cases, no.

Remember

The woman who carries an embryo not genetically related to her can nevertheless influence it, some embryonic genes will be activated and others will be silenced. She is not a passive carrier
- A specific molecule of the endometrial fluid (hsa-miR-30d) is able to reprogram the developing child by modifying embryonic gene expression. It is suspected that certain physical traits of children born by egg donation may coincide with those of the pregnant mother
- During pregnancy and parenting that lasts many years, parents and educators will impact on their children's genes for better or worse
- Parents can share their children's genetic information with their entire environment. Or with anyone. Or with the most receptive. Or only with their doctor
- There is an increase in risk of epigenetic malformations following assisted reproductive treatment. It is significant in relative terms, but quite small in absolute terms.

6. ROPA METHOD (FERTILIZED EGG TRANSFER IN FEMALE COUPLES)

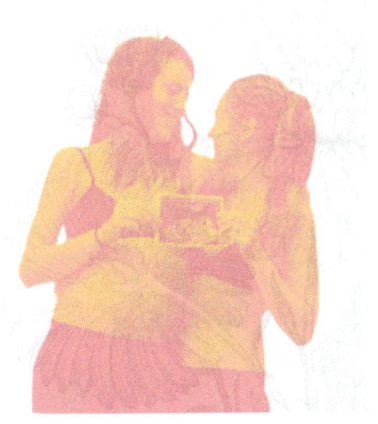

ROPA Method - Reception of Oocytes by the Partner (couple)

The ROPA (Reception of Oocytes by the Partner) method is basically an in vitro fertilization procedure between two women who come together to conceive a baby. Both women are considered mothers both biologically and legally.

One donates her eggs and the other carries the child till birth, in her pregnant belly. One contributes to the child DNA and another modulates its gene expression thanks to the exchange of information between embryo and endometrium.

The ovaries of the first woman are stimulated with hormones, followed by egg extraction in the operating room under general anesthesia and fertilized with sperm from an anonymous donor from an authorized semen bank. The embryos will spend three to five days in the laboratory to verify that they are of good quality and therefore transferable.

If all goes well, **the second woman will develop in her womb the embryo** formed with her partner's eggs and anonymous donor sperm.

Maternal instinct in a female couple

Today young lesbian women want to have children both alone and as a couple. Maternity is already included on their life horizon.

They are women of childbearing age who decide to have children through assisted reproduction centers. However, only some of the private centers in Spain provide this treatment.
This is now possible thanks to legal changes in 2006 that provided equal rights to homosexual and heterosexual patients in terms of permitted Assisted Reproduction Techniques (Law 13/2005).

Both women have the opportunity to contribute half to their own child as biological mothers, thus avoiding one of them being a simple spectator. If they want to repeat this experience so that both experience the pregnancy 'live' or to create large families, the clinic usually facilitates the the reuse of the same sperm donor for the offspring to share genetic ties.

The homoparental environment. A good parenting model

The Assisted Reproduction techniques allow the homosexual group to create new families that move away from the traditional husband and wife model, the one in which genetic, biological and legal maternity / paternity coincided.

The child who is raised by a single mother or two mothers as a couple is not disadvantaged compared to those who grow up in the traditional model of father and mother.

The family structure does not influence the development of the child, rather it will depend on education, support and as much affection as it receives, which has been associated with a higher educational level of the mother / couple of mothers.

The child who has a mother / couple of mothers who accept their homosexuality will be fortunate because they will be tolerant, brave and resilient.

Remember

The ROPA method (Reception of Oocytes by the Partner) is basically an In Vitro fertilization between two women who come together to conceive a son or daughter.
• One donates its ovarian eggs and the other carries the pregnancy in her womb to term.
Both women are considered mothers both biologically and legally
• They thus form a favorable environment for minors, like any traditional heterosexual marriage.

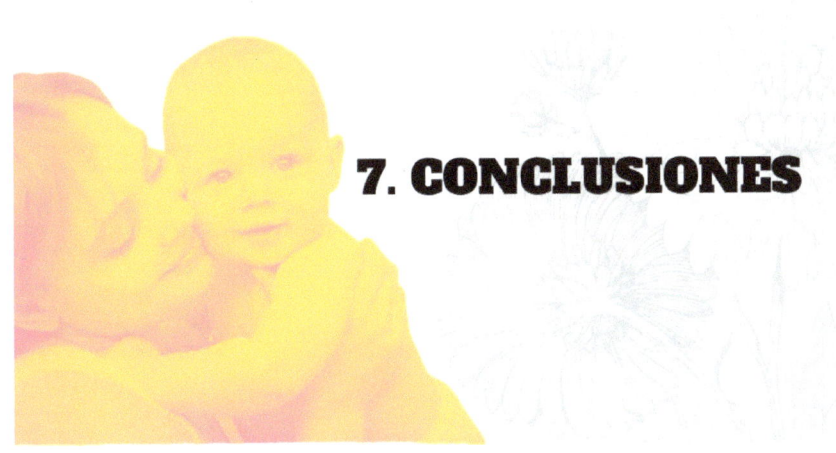

7. CONCLUSIONES

We used to believe that our character and physical features were defined only by two variables:

• by a biological (innate) factor such as genetic information that we inherit from our parents
• and by another social (acquired) factor that is the influence of the environment

That is, genetics and environment. However, epigenetics proposes a third way, it suggests that **what happens in the womb is more important than what happens after birth**.

At the time of the merger of sperm cell with an ovarian egg, the embryo carries all the genetic information not only from the father and the mother, but also from their grandparents and grandmothers. The daily life of all these people, the food they consumed, the environment in which they lived, the physical exercise they did, the chemicals they were exposed to, the positive and negative experiences they accumulated.

All of these are factors that also affect the appearance and function of our own bodies as we know them. The DNA being most sensitive to the influence of the environment at the time of conception, during the embryonic period, in childhood and puberty, these factors can exert a positive influence by activating the genes of health and silencing those of the disease. Or, vice versa a negative one by mutating the healthy genes into those predisposing to chronic endocrine, metabolic and mental dysfunction in cases of pregnant women who went through traumatic experiences, stress, violence, famine, etc.

If we understand that each person is a reflection of the genetic load invariably inherited from their parents and grandparents or grandmothers, as well as their way of life as environmental conditions that can be improved, what can we do to provide a better genetic footprint we leave on our children and grandchildren or granddaughters from the moment of conception? How can a woman receiving an ovarian egg or embryo donation reformat the genetic code of an embryo to which she is not related?

A woman can start by optimizing her fertility by clearing her body of toxins to create a healthy environment for her future baby. She can try to maintain healthy nutrition during pregnancy and lactation. She also has it in her hand to exercise moderately, reduce the episodes of stress, and above all, dedicate a lot of time, patience, and affection to her son or daughter. Time for communication, stimulation and play, time to secure attachment to the child.

Pregnant mothers should know that in any case they are active recipients of life. Even those women who have needed a gamete donation. We must not let these women down because they cannot share the usual 50% of their genetic code with their children.

Having a son or daughter is a powerful inner motor and time puts everything in its place. This boy, that girl will be her true children.

Epigenetics. The DNA of the Pregnant Mother

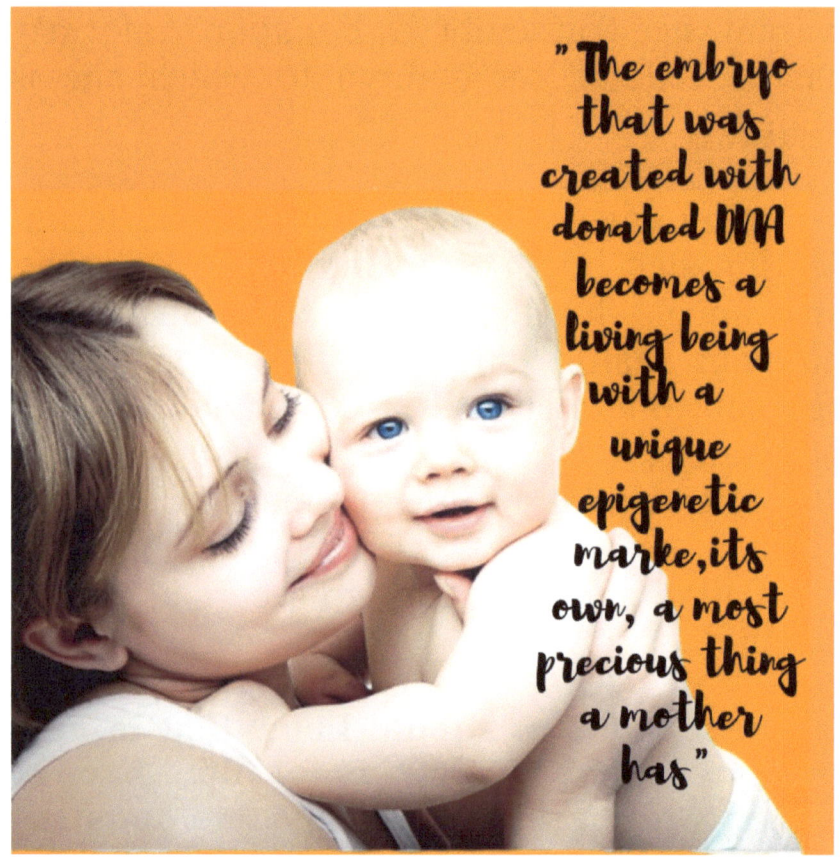

"The embryo that was created with donated DNA becomes a living being with a unique epigenetic marke, its own, a most precious thing a mother has"

8 BIBLIOGRAPHY

Inteligencia Auditiva por Victor Estalayo y rosario Vega

Bebés más inteligentes. Juegos y actividades para estimular la inteligencia del bebé por Carles Muñoz

Resiliencia por Anna Fores y Jordi Grane

Treatment of Infertility with Chinese Medicine by Jane Lyttleton

Yoga para el embarazo por Webdy Teasdill

Nutrición óptima para antes, durante y después del embarazo por Parick Holford y Susannah Lawson

Niños Adoptados por Monsterrart Lapastora y fátima Velázquez de Castro

La adopción. Una guía para padres por Carmen Barajas y otras

El niño adoptado por Keryn B. Purvis. David Cross. Wendy Lyons Sunshine

Integral por Colin Campbell y Howard Jacobs

http://www.antena3.com/noticias/salud/embarazada-puede-modificar-genetica-hijo_20150923571792064beb281757e4fdc2.html

https://ivi.es/blog/epigenetica-un-nuevo-hallazgo-que-demuestra-la-comunicacion-entre-la-futura-madre-y-su-embrion/

https://ivi.es/notas/una-investigacion-sobre-epigenetica-abre-la-puerta-a-la-detencion-de-la-transmision-de-enfermedades-como-diabetes-y-obesidad/

LICENSE

The license to use this e-book **Creative Commons Attribution Non-Commercial-ShareAlike 4.0 International (CC BY-NC-SA 4.0)** is only for your personal use and enjoyment. Because of this, you can not plagiarize it in whole or in part, resell it or illegally download it, or give it to others without the author's permission. If you want to share it, kindly purchase a copy. Thank you for respecting the author's hard work.

TEXT, COVER AND MAKING OF THE E-BOOK BY SARA TOLEDO

Free cover image for commercial use courtesy of www.flickr.com Madrid 2017

ENGLISH TRANSLATION BY GIORAH BEN SHAUL

Madrid 2.020

CONTENT

1. EPIGENETICS: INTRODUCTION

Hungry and pregnant. Holland, 1944........3

What is epigenetics?...............................7

The environment also has an influence.....9

Remember..10

2. WILL MY GENES SHOW UP?

Genetic inheritance is not something completely given 11

Physical Features………………………….11

Intelligence (high capacities).............................12

Diseases………………………………….12

Epimutations...13

Remember..15

3. DETRIMENTAL EPIGENETIC MEMORY

    Genetic sensitivity..............................16

    A) About embryo..............................17

    B) Chilhood and puberty 19

    Remember.......................................21

4. GENES FOR HEALTH

    From Health Genes to Illness Genes...23

    Nutrition and maternal womb 25

    10 daily routines that reformat your baby's DNA inside your uterus.....................25

    Reproductive health.........................39

    A) Nutrients....................................39

    B) Antinutrients..............................41

    Remember.......................................44

5. EPIGENETICS IN ASSISTED REPRODUCTION

Road start (Kilometer 0): I am infertile..46

Active reception of ovarian eggs. You are not a passive mom...............................47

The pregnant mother does contribute. Exchange between endometrium and embryo..49

A possibility of transmitting physical features or cognitive and character traits of the pregnant mother to the next generation?..52

Similar and not by chance.....................59

The personality of the children does not depend on egg donation........................60

To tell or to keep quiet in the larger family..61

Anonymous vs known donor?................62

Do Assisted Reproduction Techniques (ART) leave an epigenetic mark?............63

Remember..64

6. ROPA METHOD (FERTILIZED EGG TRANSFER IN FEMALE COUPLES)

ROPA Method - Reception of Oocytes by the Partner (couple)..............................65

Maternal instinct in a female couple....66

The homoparental environment. A good parenting model......................................67

Remember..68

7. CONCLUSIONS..69
8. BIBLIOGRAPHY.......................................73

www.ingramcontent.com/pod-product-compliance
Lightning Source LLC
Chambersburg PA
CBHW041103180526
45172CB00001B/89